Wilderness Survival Mistakes:
25 Mistakes That Will Cost Your Life

Table of content

Introduction

Going out on some amazing trips and camps is very exciting. It is probably one of the best things that a person can do during his stay on this planet. But with every enjoyment there are certain hardships and it is our duty to be fully aware about all these hardships and prepare ourselves. We need to know about all the dangers and all the things which can put our life in danger. We should know and prepare ourselves so we can be able to tackle all the different situations that come in our life. There are fair chances for any person to get lost in the woods. You obviously do not intend to get lost but anything can happen. One should prepare himself for any situation to occur. There are quite a few people who understand how important it is to consider the fact that being prepared for anything and every situation is very necessary. Never be a hundred percent sure that you will return no matter what happens.

So in order to let our readers know about the different dangers and things that can make you more prone to lose your life, this book has been written with all the different mistakes that play a major role in putting your life in danger. This book tells you about all the different mistakes that can make you one step closer to losing your life in the wild.

Chapter 1 – Never lose hope when lost in the Wild

People often give up when they find themselves lost in the woods. One thing that should be understood by every person is that you always maximum chances of survival no matter how bad the situation is. So never lose hope. There have been many cases which have been reported and the reason why people had lesser chances of survival was loss of hope and panic. So in order to save yourself you need to remember that you should make lesser mistakes and increase the good choices that you make.

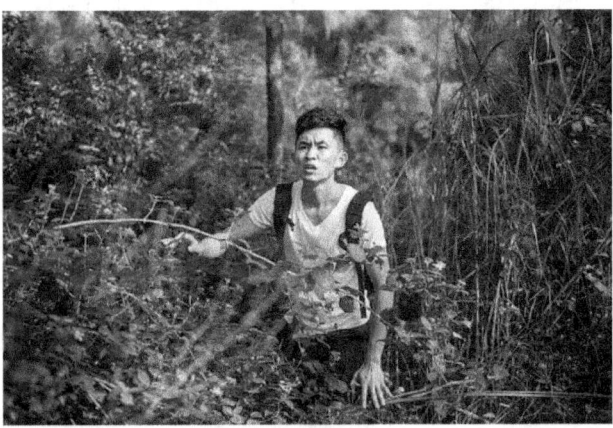

There is no other way through which you can help yourself and save yourself from all the hardships that you will be facing in the wild. You need to set your priorities. You need to know what right and what's wrong when you are out alone. You need to keep every single thing in your mind and be aware of the things happening around you. You need to all those things that are required in order to be safe and sound in the wild. Some of the things that will help you build up all the hope that you need are as follows:

Be calm

The most important thing that people forget to maintain is their level of calmness. You need to remember that no matter what you need to remain calm in order to maintain your sanity. People often lose their minds just because they panic to an extent that no person can help them come back to the normal state. You need to remain calm in order to avoid any further dangers and inconveniences. You need to remember that the more you remain out raged and panicked in the whole situation there is a clear chances that you will decrease the chances of your survival. You will lose all hope that is in you. You won't be able to think clearly and save your life from obvious dangers that are coming up. So in order to get all the hope inside you, you need to remain calm.

Look out for obvious lifesaving items

When you are lost in the wild there are certain things which can save your life. But because of all the trauma and stress which you go through, you often fail to see and discover those things and ultimately come to the conclusion that you will not survive this incident. You need to remember that there are things which are sure to help you out. You just need to open your mind and think clearly. Look for things that can help you save your life and live a better and prosperous life ahead. This can only be done if you know how to judge and find the things which are going to save your life. Look out for sources of water and food. You need to know the limit for which you can live without food and without water. You can live much longer without food as compared to water so never compromise on the water intake that you have even in the wild because this will lead to a direct compromise on your life.

Safe place

Most important matter even than food and water that needs special attention in the wild is a safe place to stay. When you get lost in the wild to get to face any such circumstance, don't just go out and search for water and food in the first place. You need to remember that you still have time even if you don't find water for several hours. But before it gets dark you need to remember that you cannot survive without shelter. You need to find shelter no matter what and this should be your priority. People who simply get out and start finding food and water tend to have lesser chances of survival because they neglect how important it is to have shelter in order to be safe. So get your stuff and sources ready for a safe place to stay till you are found and this is very important as there are chances that when it gets dark it might get even harder for you to find a safe and sound place for yourself.

Water over food

Always remember that you can survive much longer without food as compared to water. So whenever you get lost, searching for water should be your priority. You need to find water first and then food and other solid items to eat. There are many places where you can find water. You should look around and observe the different areas that are close to you and search for a source of water. If you think that there is no water available in the area where you are searching then you need to chance your technique. You can always go to lower areas because water is a liquid and liquid always moves along the force of gravity. So there are fair chances that you will find water content in the lower areas of land. You just have to look out for the right places.

Chapter 2 – Five of the most life threatening mistakes

Technically speaking there are hundreds of mistakes that people make when they get lost. And it is these mistakes which can lead to reduced chances of their survival. To help people get out of this problem this chapter is focusing on the five most commonly made mistakes which every person should avoid if they find themselves lost into the wild. These five mistakes are those mistakes which are the most common and most deadly hence should be avoided at all costs. There are obviously many other reason and mistakes as well but in this chapter we will be talking about the most common ones only.

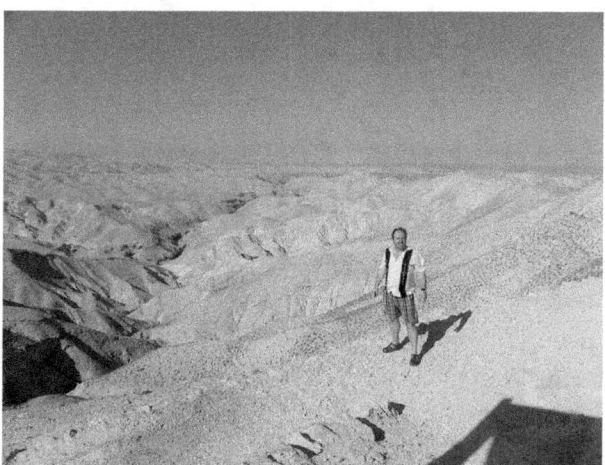

Mistake 1: Roof over your head

Many people who have reported to be lost and ended up with losing all their chances of survival reported that one of the most important and very basic mistake which many people make at the time of such emergency and panicking situation is that they fail to understand the importance of a roof over their head where they can spend their days and nights. This is something that many people fail to understand and instead start looking out for things other than shelter like food and water. No doubt, water and food are also a very important but finding a shelter is even more important than everything else. What people generally do is that first they start panicking. Then once they have regained their sanity finally, they begin searching for things other than shelter. As a result of this, the night arrives and now they fail to find a proper place where they can spend their night. Many times, the weather in the wild is so extreme that it can lead to fatal conditions. People often fail to survive in the harsh weather and end up losing their life because of this mistake.

Mistake 2: Not having all the essential tools

One of the most important things that people fail to understand is the importance of all those tools that can help you understand where you are. That can tell you the place and direction to where you are heading. These information's might seem to be very silly and petty to you at the moment but when a person is lost, people understand the true value of all these tools. The most important thing to be kept in mind is that these things will help you to get back or head in the right direction. You need to understand that how important these things are if you want to go into the right direction. So whenever you head to any place with the intent of enjoying and sightseeing always keep the essential tools which will help you and guide you to the right direction. In case you accidently end up being in such a situation like a crash or any other unforeseen circumstance then you should always remember that things like seeing where the sun rises and sets can always give you an idea about the direction so keep your eyes open and be alert.

Mistake 3: Not being prepared

Another very important and very common mistake made by many people is that they often underestimate and fail to understand about the task and trip which they are going to make. They think that going out in the wild is going to be a piece of cake and no preparation is needed for it. In case you don't know, but knowing some of the very basic techniques and ideas of camping is very important. Every person should be aware of how they should survive in harsh and difficult conditions. Every person should understand the importance of having the right information with them no matter how able they think of themselves. You never know what might come in handy. So learn about some of the very basic things like how to signal in case you get lost or stranded, how to build a roof for yourself from things that are available in front of you at that moment, what are the options of things that are edible in the wild and how you can search for other items in the wild. All of these things will come from practice and right preparation.

Mistake 4: inappropriate clothing

Now comes another very important mistake made by many travelers around the world. Sometimes people who go out into the wild wear clothes that are not warm enough thinking that it is going to be pretty hot. But technically speaking, there is a rule of thumb which applies here. This rule suggests that just when you think that the clothes that you have on are enough, wear another layer of clothing. If you think that wearing more clothes sounds absurd then hear this. If at any point you think that you feel hot and cannot bear the temperature, you can always take off the extra article of clothing which you are wearing and keep it aside. But if you leave your clothes at home and don't have anything to wear then you are sure to put your life in danger.

Mistake 5: underestimating the dangers

People who make spontaneous never look and think over the risk factors which they have to face. This is something which leads to poor survival rates. Just by sitting with a couple of your friends and thinking about spontaneously getting ready for some place is obviously going to chaos because in such situations you do not have the right plans and calculations of things in your mind. Always plan what you are going to do.

Chapter 3 – Ten common mistakes while surviving in the woods

This chapter focuses on the ten most common mistakes which are made by many people when they get lost and survive in the woods alone. The purpose of this chapter is to make people aware and let them know how to avoid these mistakes by knowing them beforehand.

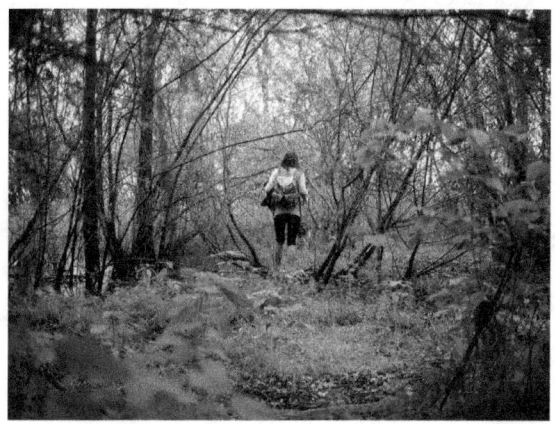

Mistake 1:

A very common mistake made by people who get lost is that they fail to understand the importance of drinking safe and potable water. We do understand that when a person gets lost, and stays in the wild for longer periods of time, then getting any type and source of water seems to be a blessing. But one thing that many people fail to understand is that in order to stay alive, you need to drink safe and potable water. If you drink water which is contaminated, you are sure to get diseases that will also lead to you death due to dehydration.

Mistake 2:

Another very common mistake is that people often forget that they need to make other people aware that they are stuck in the wild. They need to let the world know regarding their presence and this cannot be possible if you do not know about the tricks which are required to make signal your presence in the woods. So to make people know, you should firstly have all the essential survival tools that help you know how to get out of the woods and indicate your presence. And in case you do not have any of those you should be aware of the ways in which you can signal your presence.

Mistake 3:

There have been cases where people who get lost do not opt for creating fire in their vicinity. There are several reasons as to why they do so. Some do not know how to build a fire where as others are scared of how will they manage the fire which they will create and some find it as a source of potential danger. The main thing which should be kept in mind is that fire will always help you save yourself from a number of different dangers in one way or another.

Mistake 4:

You must have already heard about the fact that taking short cuts can often lead to even more dangers in one's life. You need to understand that never go for the routes or ways that might seem short to you and a little dangerous. Don't go for such ideas just for the sake of getting to a place earlier. The reason is that it often leads to unforeseen circumstances which eventually lead to death.

Mistake 5:

Some people think that water which is found in the streams or any other source can be used as it is without purifying it. In order to keep yourself safe from diseases and other problems you should always purify the water which you drink. There are a number of different ways in which this can be done. People who come prepared for any situation often carry tablets for purifying water. Besides this, boiling water can always be the best source.

Mistake 6:

There are many cases where people often fail to understand the importance of planning a trip. If you think that you are already at a trip and you further want to increase the duration of the trip where you are then you are extremely mistaken. When you stay longer than what you have planned, there are chances that people often do not have enough supplies as they do not intend to stay for longer period of time. So always limit your stay to what has been planned instead of prolonging it too much longer durations.

Mistake 7:

A very common mistake that is done by many travelers is that once they find out and realize that they are lost, they still continue to move from place to place instead of staying at one place. It is human nature that most of the people think that if they keep moving ahead they might lead themselves to the right path. But this is not the case every time. You should always stop and camp when you find yourself lost and get a roof over your head.

Mistake 8:

Another very common yet understandable mistake is that people forget to remain calm. You need to remember that no matter happens you should keep your state of mind and level at the right place. You should remember that without having an alert and conscious mind you can never save yourself from any calamity. So keep yourself active and alert at all times to save yourself from the risks of being in danger.

Mistake 9:

When you go on trips you need to remember that no matter how lazy you might be at home, this is no place to be lazy. Always remember that no matter what happens you are supposed to be active and energetic while you are in the wild.

Mistake 10:

People often end up making a common mistake of camping in lower areas. Always camp on areas that are high above. This way you are sure of the things and areas that are below. You do not have any danger or risk of things that might fall upon you because you are the only one who's on top.

Chapter 4 – Ten mistake to avoid while alone in the wild

To increase your knowledge and chances of survival in the wild, here are ten more mistakes that you should avoid when you find yourself alone and stranded in the woods. These mistakes are sure to cost you your life if not treated and avoided accordingly.

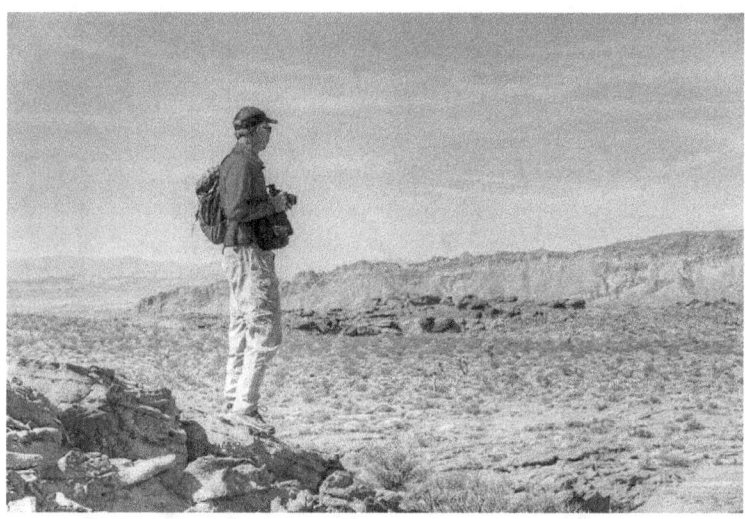

Mistake 1:

When people go out for camping in the wild, they often think that having a mere shelter on their head will be enough for them but in reality this sis not enough if they want to protect themselves from the wild animals and other calamities. The most important thing that many people fail to perform is to manage how they can set the boundaries which may act as a hindrance for other creatures and dangers.

Mistake 2:

A very common mistake made by many travelers and campers is that they ignore some of the most important signs. If you think that weather forecast and the current weather conditions indicate a tough weather then you need to be aware and keep yourself in a safe position. Don't take these warning too lightly. If you think that there is going to be rain and heavy flooding in the area that you have camped, then it is your duty to move to areas which are high up in order to save your lives no matter how hard it is.

Mistake 3:

If you ever get into a situation where you think that you are lost, don't ever make the mistake of simply sitting in one place and doing nothing just waiting for someone to come and rescue. Never make this mistake. You need to get up and look around the area where you are at. Look around and see what is around you so that you become familiar with the surroundings. It is very important to understand that in order to increase your chances of survival you should be well aware of the area where you are at. You should about all the different things which are around you so that you understand about your risks and chances of survival.

Mistake 4:

In case you have made a plan for going out in the wild, you need to learn the basic skills and techniques that every traveler and camper should be aware of. You should be aware of the basic skills that will help you survive the harsh environment like how to stalk, how to kill and slaughter some basic animals, ways through which you can store the things you get whether it is food items or other things etc.

Mistake 5:

A very common mistake made by many traveler and campers is that they are never prepared for the worst conditions. Once you set out for a camp or any other trip you should always have a separate plan which is supposed to guide you and tell you about how you can find your way back to the surface. What are the ways through which you can get yourself out of the dangerous situation? Always leave your houses with a plan which can help you survive in the emergency situation.

Mistake 6:

When people leave for trips and camps, they keep a certain amount of food. A very common   mistake that is made by almost everyone is that they do not keep sufficient amount of food with themselves. They think that the food which they have kept is going to be enough for them when this is not the actual case. There are cases in which people fail to keep sufficient food for themselves which will help them survive for longer periods of time. So in order o save yourself form any hardship always keep more food than what you think is going to be enough for you.

Mistake 7:

Whenever you leave out for a camp or head any way into the wild, always remember that even if you intent to keep yourself away from the people and disconnected from what you have in the world, you still need to have something that can help you stay connected to the world. Always remember to keep the important gadgets with you even if you start your journey with the intent of staying away from people for a little while. This surely does not mean that you leave all the things behind at home.

Mistake 8:

If we start thinking about things that are important and might help you get through the most difficult situations, then there are many. But a very important and handy item that is sure to help you in case you get lost is duct tape. Leaving duct tape behind will the most stupid mistake that you can ever do before going on a trip. It can save you from so many disasters.

Mistake 9:

In case you find yourself lost in the woods the most important thing which is to be done in this case is to save all the encouragement and positivity in you. You need to remember that this is not the end of the world. People who lose all their hope and motivation are sure to get into danger.

Mistake 10:

The most common mistake that should be noted is never pack a lot things. Don't pack things that you might not even use. Be aware of all the things that you might use and those which are important. Don't just keep on stuffing your bags with unnecessary things.

Chapter 5 – Important life hacks in the wild

When a person gets into an unforeseen situation, chances are that you don't understand what you are supposed to do. Instead you might ruin the chances of your survival. So in this chapter there are a few things which will help you get better chances of survival.

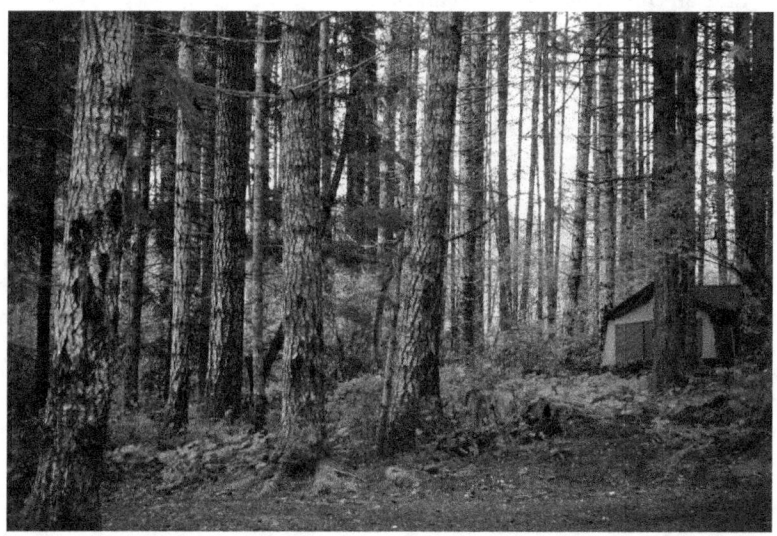

The first and foremost step

The first thing that any person should do once he finds himself stranded in the woods is to get some fire started out. This is very important and major step. This will help you with a lot of things. By building a fire you will save yourself from the extreme weather condition during the night. You will save yourself from feeling cold. So start some fire in order to keep yourself warm. If you think that you are stuck in a situation where the weather is warm and you do not require fire then remember that fire is not only used in order to make yourself warm. When the night sets in it is going to get darker. Staying in the dark when you are in the woods can be frightening. If you get some fire started you are sure to create some light in the area where you are. This will make you feel comfortable and safe if nothing else.

Gather all the wood that you can find

The first thing you need to remember is to get lots of wood. Wood is never enough. You never know what kind of trees and wood is present in the area where you are at. There are certain woods that get consumed much faster than the rest. Then there are those which take longer time in order to turn into ashes. So to help you survive through the entire night you should be sure that you have enough wood with yourself. Now the question is how do you know that you have got enough fire with you? a very good rule that is applied in most of the cases is that when you set out to get the wood for your fire and when you think that the amount of wood which you have gathered is enough and sufficient then you should go out again and get at least three more piles of wood which are just the same as the one which you got before. This is the amount of wood that is actually enough for you to spend your whole night.

Items that can be used other than wood

There are different types of things which can be used when you are getting a fire started. If you use wood only as a source of fire that is also fine. In case you want to use fire that can create more and more smoke which will save you and let others know that there is someone in the woods then you should trying adding different things in the fire that will create more smoke. A few examples of things that can be used are brush, wood that is green and boughs of trees. You can also use dung if you find any.

Look for what you are starting

Another very important thing to be kept in mind is the size of the fire you start. You need to remember that once you are starting the fire and have got all the materials which are necessary to start it, you should always be conscious about the size of the fire which you start. If you start a small fire which is small, you should know that it will be more than enough for you. You are going to face a lot of difficulties if you think that having a bigger fire is going to be helpful because it's not. First thing is that you are going to need a lot of wood in order to maintain a bigger fire. So keep it as small as you can. Secondly you will be wasting a lot of time in order to keep that fire running and starting it in the first place.

Be sure about the safety of your surrounding area

When you start fire, you should always make sure that it is in an area where you can control the fire which you have started. Look around and find a safe place to get your fire started. There are going to be a lot of things and factors which might aggravate the conditions and worsen everything. Don't start a fire near trees, plants or any brush that you think might catch fire. This is going to put you in a lot of danger. There are chances that you might set the entire forest into fire. When you are trying to maintain the fire you should always monitor and see if you are giving in enough wood. You don't want to put in a lot of wood in the fire so that it gets bigger. You also need to see the weather conditions of the place you are at. See how to manage the fire according to the weather and the wind that blows.

23

Conclusion

There is absolutely no way that you are a hundred percent ready for every situation that comes to you. There are always those chances in which you might lose your life when you in the wild. There is no assurance that you will return without being harmed from the woods. The question here is that are you prepared for the worst? Do you know that to do and what not to do in the wild? This book consists of twenty five different mistakes that people often make when they set out in the wild. They are often not aware of the many hardships that will come in their way if they fail to perform some very important and basic techniques.

This book has given you all the detail about the things which should be done in the wild and things which should not be done. It has given you the detail of the most important and common twenty five mistakes that can cost your life while you are in the wild. Now it's your job to understand the significance and delicacy of these mistakes and stop making them whenever you go out again in the wild. Hope you enjoyed your read!

FREE Bonus Reminder

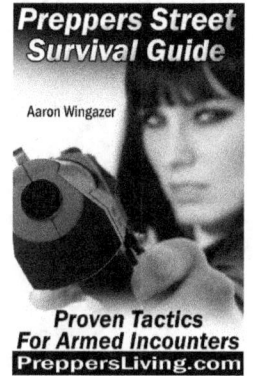

If you have not grabbed it yet, please go ahead and download your special bonus report
"Preppers Street Survival Guide: Proven Tactics For Armed Incounters"

SimplyClicktheButtonBelow

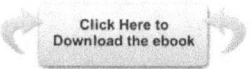

OR **Go to This Page**

http://preppersliving.com/free

BONUS #2: More Free & Discounted Books & Products

Do you want to receive more Free/Discounted Books or Products?

We have a mailing list where we send out our new Books or Products when they go free or with a discount on Amazon. Click on the link below to sign up for Free & Discount Book & Product Promotions.

=> Sign Up for Free & Discount Book & Product Promotions <=

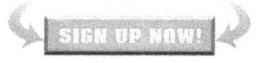

OR Go to this URL

http://zbit.ly/1WBb1Ek